Making Herbal Dream Pillows

JIM LONG

Illustrated by Dagmar Fehlau

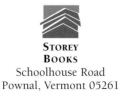

STOREY BOOKS
Schoolhouse Road
Pownal, Vermont 05261

8593758

The mission of Storey Communications is to serve our customers
by publishing practical information that encourages personal independence
in harmony with the environment.

Dedication

To Jerry Stamps, who first introduced me to dream pillows;
Billy Joe Tatum, for her enthusiasm, inspiration, and guidance;
Joshua Young, who always believes in me, encourages my projects, and makes my writing possible;
and my children, Lori Marie and Traci Lynn, who are always in my dreams.

Edited by Deborah Balmuth and Robin Catalano
Cover design by Meredith Maker
Text design by E.K Weymouth Design
Production assistance by Susan Bernier
Illustrations by Dagmar Fehlau
Line drawings by Helen Long

Printed in Hong Kong by C & C Offset Printing Co Ltd.
10 9 8 7 6 5 4 3 2 1

Library of Congress Cataloging-in-Publication Data

Long, Jim, 1946–
   Making Herbal Dream Pillows
     p.   cm. — (The spirit of aromatherapy)
   ISBN 1-58017-075-7 (alk. paper)
   1. Aromatherapy.   2. Herbs — Therapeutic use.
   3. Potpourris (Scented floral mixtures)   4. Dreams.
   5. Sleep.   I. Title.   II. Series.
RM666.A68L66   1998
615'. 321 — dc21   98-14498
                          CIP

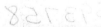

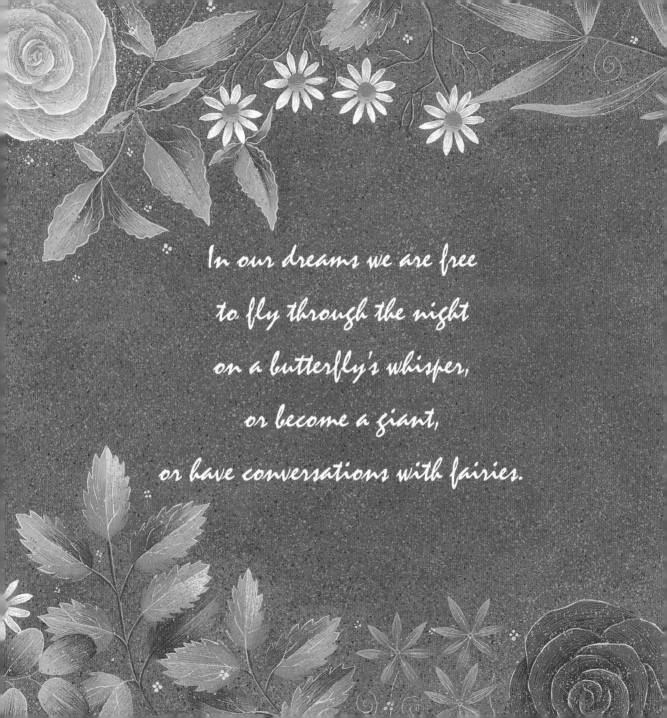

In our dreams we are free
to fly through the night
on a butterfly's whisper,
or become a giant,
or have conversations with fairies.

Contents

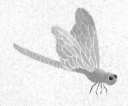

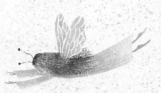

The Origins of Dream Pillows

The European craft of making dream pillows goes back several centuries.

Dream pillows recall a time in our history when people assigned magical powers to herbs.

Certain herbs under the pillow were believed to protect against evil, foretell the future,

or conjure up lovers. Ancient stories tell of herbs that were used to calm bad dreams,

bring about good dreams, or quiet the restless sleeper.

Modern reasoning tells us that herbs can't predict events or ward off evil.

However, there is much evidence, both historical and modern, that pleasant fragrances

from herbs and flowers do have a positive effect on dreaming. Considerable research

in the area of aromatherapy demonstrates that the fragrances of certain herbs and flowers

enable us to relax, while other fragrances can cause workers to be more alert

on the job and students in the classroom to remain awake.

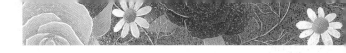

Comfort Pillows

Dream pillows were once called comfort pillows, and were used in the sickroom to ease the nightmares that may come with medicine and the smells of illness. Relaxing herbs — primarily catnip, lavender, and mugwort — combined in little pillows were respected for their usefulness in easing the sleep of crying babies.

I first learned about dream pillows from a pharmacist. He had gotten his degree from a respected school of pharmacy, but as a boy had also studied with an old gentleman pharmacist who was very knowledgeable about herbs and called himself an apothecary.

I went to the pharmacist to get a prescription filled for some medicine to help me sleep. I was struggling with a difficult divorce, and had spent sleepless nights worrying about the welfare of my children. When sleep did come, it was filled with nightmares and restlessness.

The pharmacist, who was also a friend, had heard me say before that I took medication only as absolutely necessary, preferring alterna-

tives when available. So when I gave him the prescription for the sleeping medicine, he quickly offered another possibility.

"I think you'd do better with a dream pillow and a mild relaxing herb," he said.

He handed me a bottle of valerian capsules and a little cloth pillow, about three inches wide and five inches long, stuffed with something soft and tied with a string. They would would help me relax, he explained, allowing, but not causing, sleep.

"Take three valerian capsules about thirty minutes before you go to bed, and place this little pillow in your pillowcase and leave it there," he instructed. "There aren't any bad side effects. If this doesn't help, come back and I'll fill your prescription."

I'd never heard of dream pillows back then, but I followed his advice. Within ten days I was sleeping better, having fewer nightmares, and was more able to make plans and decisions. I put the dream pillow out of my mind, crediting the power of suggestion for my improved sleep.

Dreams with a Twist

It was about five years later that I had my second encounter with a dream pillow. I was staying with friends in Arkansas while I was overseeing the construction of a public garden. The friends' home had a guest room upstairs, with a single bed that was surrounded by lots of little pillows. I would stay at their house for four or five days at a time, go home for a weekend, and return again to their home during the week.

I've always been an active dreamer, but in their house my dreams took on a different twist. At home on weekends I dreamed peacefully and normally, but during the week I repeatedly had horrible, colorfully terrorizing nightmares. Several mornings at breakfast I would begin conversation with, "I have to tell you about the awful dream I had last night."

One morning another friend heard me relating the past night's dream. "Oh, I always have gruesome nightmares when I sleep in that room," she said.

Our host said, "I'll bet there's a dream pillow up there in one of the pillows," and after breakfast we went up to check. Within minutes my host pulled a little cloth pillow out of one of the larger decorative pillows.

She took the little bag downstairs and emptied out the contents onto a newspaper. With her finger she began moving the ingredients around on the paper, describing what she found. "Here are pungent French marigold blossoms, and here is a bay leaf. Look, here's tansy, even some Russian tarragon. Good grief, no wonder you were having nightmares. This isn't a dream mix at all. Someone has mistakenly filled a dream bag with a bunch of moth-repelling herbs. These herbs shouldn't ever be used in a dream blend!"

I was impressed both at the intensity of dreams I'd had and at the fact that I had not known the pillow was there at all, but I certainly had experienced a marked change in my dreaming.

Scent Connects You with Memories

Within a few weeks I began researching dream pillows, looking at herbals dating back two and three centuries. I learned that dream pillows are based on the way fragrances elicit memories in our brain. I found that certain smells can arouse a memory that was long forgotten. The smell of roses can conjure up a favorite aunt not thought about since childhood. A whiff of perfume sensed on a busy street corner can bring a memory, in a flash, of that first date in high school. The part of our brains where memory is stored responds to our sense of smell, seemingly faster than to most of our other senses.

I began looking at old formulas for dream blends in antique books, reading anything written, ancient and modern, and began to get a sense of what kinds of herbs and flowers were believed to cause different kinds of dreams. With my growing research I started preparing dream blends for specific kinds of dreams, then trying them out on myself and friends.

Over the years I have formulated dozens of dream blends and come up with lists of herbs and flowers that encourage particular kinds of dreams when used in a variety of combinations.

Dream blends are *very* different from potpourri; do not expect a dream blend to have the noticeable strong smells of a potpourri blend. Dream blends are subtle. Their fragrances are released as you move about on the pillow during sleep. For most people, dream blends bring about a change in dreaming, add color to black and white dreams, or quiet restless sleep. Most of all, herbal dream pillows are a pleasant way to promote creative dreaming and more restful sleep.

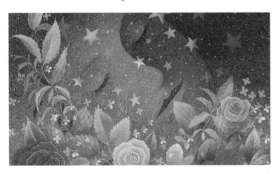

Herbs to Avoid

Artemisia (except for mugwort) should be avoided, as many kinds of artemisia can cause frightening dreams and, after waking, headaches.

Bay, which sometimes causes headaches upon waking, can also add a gray-brown color and violent quality to dreams.

Fixatives are not recommended for use in dream blends. These include cellulose (processed corncobs) and orrisroot. Since they contain some fragrance they may change the texture of the dream blend, making the results unpredictable. Orrisroot can also cause headaches upon waking.

Oils of any kind are not recommended. Oils are highly concentrated and can overpower other herbs.

Russian tarragon can cause frightening nightmares.

Sage can create a haunting feeling in dreams. However, garden sage blossoms and clary sage blossoms can be used in small amounts in dream blends.

Tansy, which can cause violent and terrifying nightmares, can also produce headaches upon waking.

Plants in the Herbal Dream Garden

Many types of plants can be used in herbal dream pillows, but here are some of the most common and versatile.

Aniseed

(*Pimpinella anisum*). *Curtin's Healing Herbs of the Rio Grande* suggests that in folklore the fragrance of aniseed keeps men from dreaming. It's useful in relaxing blends.

Balsam fir

(*Abies balsamea*). Fir needles are a pleasant addition to relaxing blends, good in combination with lavender, hops, and roses. They impart an outdoors feeling to dreams.

Calendula

(*Calendula officinalis*). In folklore it is said that combining sage and calendula blossoms will make dreams come true. Calendula, in small amounts, can add restfulness to a blend, and moderate more spicy ingredients.

Catnip

(*Nepeta cataria*). This herb has been used for centuries to ease babies' troubled sleep. Today, we use it in adult blends to induce relaxation and sleep.

Chamomile

(*Matricaria chamomilla*). Chamomile is used for relaxation and pleasant dreams. People who are allergic to ragweed should probably avoid using this herb in their blends, as it sometimes causes similar reactions.

Cinnamon

(*Cinnamomum zeylanicum*). Cinnamon has recently been proved by fragrance researchers to be one of the most erotic aromas for men. Cinnamon comes from the bark of a tropical evergreen tree. Use it sparingly in dream blends for an exotic, romantic texture.

Cloves

(*Syzygium aromaticum*). Cloves add a hint of spiciness, especially when used with roses in romantic mixes, but use them sparingly: Just 3 or 4 cloves in a blend is plenty.

Hops

(*Humulus lupulus*). This herb is actually the flower from a perennial vine and there are several varieties, including some considered "bitter" and others "sweet." Sweet hop flowers are the ones used for dreaming; they induce relaxation and peacefulness.

Jasmine

(*Jasminum officinale* or *J. odoratissimum*). The delicious fragrance of jasmine will almost encourage dreaming when you're awake! The dried flowers lend an exotic and romantic feeling to dreams, especially for women.

Lavender

(*Lavandula* spp.). Lavender aids in easing headaches when you are awake, and is useful in relaxing blends alone or in combination with roses and mugwort. Combined with jasmine and roses, lavender adds warmth and familiarity to romantic mixes.

Leather

While it seems an unlikely ingredient, leather is tanned with a product that comes from oak bark. The scent of fresh leather trimmings adds excitement and energy to dream blends.

Lemon balm

(Melissa officinalis). In aromatherapy, lemon balm is used to relieve depression, anxiety, insomnia, and nervous tension. This herb combines well with roses, lavender, thyme, hops, and mint. A mix of lemon balm and lavender, in equal parts, is useful in relieving headache and stress.

Lemongrass

(Cymbopogon citratus). A native herb of tropical regions, lemongrass adds a bit of color and a soothingly safe, mildly exotic feeling to blends.

Lemon verbena

(Aloysia triphylla). Native to Chile and Argentina, this shrub produces delightfully aromatic leaves that can add a bit of lightness, even feelings of flying, to the dream blend when used in small amounts.

Lilac

(Syringa chinensis). Use lilac for sweet, safe, and peaceful dream mixes, in small amounts. It's also good in mixes for the sickroom, and for travelers' blends. In larger amounts, lilac adds sensuality.

Marjoram, Sweet

(Origanum majorana). Sweet marjoram is often used in blends to ease nervousness and restlessness during sleep. I find that this herb adds a dimension of warmth, safety, and comfort to dreams.

Mimosa flowers

(Acacia dealbata). Somewhat like jasmine, only milder, mimosa can add an exotic, more complex feeling to dreams. Mimosa and lemon balm are a good combination for peaceful but slightly colorful dreaming.

Mint

(Mentha spp.). Just a small amount of mint works like a tuning knob on a television: It adds clarity, vividness, and color to dreams.

Mugwort

(Artemisia vulgaris). In folklore it is said that this herb causes the dreamer to remember his or her dreams. It does seem to increase clarity, while also encouraging relaxation.

Passionflower

(Passiflora incarnata). Used as a mild sedative in herbal medicines, passionflower adds a quieting effect to the dream pillow. Flowers and leaves are both used, but flowers are preferred.

Rose

(Rosa spp.). Rose petals create a feeling of loving thoughts and warmth. Used with more exotic herbs in romantic or adventurous mixes, roses keep the feeling of the dream grounded in safety and peacefulness.

Rosemary

(Rosmarinum officinalis). In folklore, rosemary was used to ensure sleep and keep away bad dreams. Rosemary works well with a bit of lavender, roses, mugwort, and hops for a relaxing night's sleep without notable dreaming.

Thyme

(Thymus spp.). Herb lore of old claims that sleeping on a pillow of thyme allows the dreamer to see fairies. I generally combine thyme with roses, hops, lavender, and rosemary for a peaceful, quiet dream.

Mixing the Dream Blend

A dream blend consists of carefully selected herbs, flowers, needles, or leaves that are combined and then allowed to sit overnight — in a closed container — so the fragrances blend. Place the mixture in the cloth of your choice; sew up the end, and you're ready to use your pillow. It's that simple!

Selecting the Herbs and Flowers

The very best herbs for your dream blends are those that you grow yourself; you will know they're fresh and pesticide-free. If you can't grow your own, buy your dried ingredients from a reputable grower who uses organic methods.

From healthy plants choose whole leaves, flowers, needles, and other parts as described in the dream blend recipes. Be sure you are selecting only ingredients that have not been sprayed with chemicals.

Microwave Drying

I never recommend drying herbs in the microwave. That method actually explodes the fragrant oil cells of the plant and removes most of the scent and flavor of the herb, leaving you with a tasteless, and thus fragrance-less, piece of greenery.

Preparing the Herbs and Flowers

Pick the herbs or flowers in midday, after the dew has evaporated. Don't wash the herbs; washing removes some of the fragrant oils. If there is soil clinging to the leaves, shake the herbs or rub them between your fingers.

Place the herbs on the shelves of a food dehydrator and dry on lowest heat setting until they are crisp. Or, rubber band the herbs in small bunches and hang them in a warm, airy, dark place. When dry, store in airtight plastic containers or zipper bags, in a dark place, until ready to use.

You can also put the herbs loosely in a paper bag, or on a cookie sheet and place that in the trunk of the car on a hot day. Remove the herbs as soon as they are crisp and dry (about one or two days), then store in airtight containers in a dark place.

Blending the Herbs and Flowers

Choose the dream blend you want to create. Assemble all of the ingredients listed, in the amounts indicated, and place them together in a plastic zipper bag. Stir or shake to mix the ingredients, seal, and put them away for 24 to 48 hours to let the fragrances blend.

Creating the Dream Pillow

The dream pillow is a small bag or pillow made of cloth and filled with herbs. The bag or pillow is tucked inside your pillowcase. The herbs will be crushed slightly as your head moves about during sleep. As the herbs are crushed, they release their subtle aromas.

Materials

one 5" by 12" strip of fabric

one handful cotton batting or fiberfill

½ cup dream blend

1. For a decorative pillow, choose a piece of cloth that is attractive and fits the theme of the blend you are using (a flowered cloth for romance, for example, or boldly colored material for creativity). Cotton, a natural fabric, is preferred over synthetics.

2. Cut out a piece of cloth that is 5" by 12". Fold it in half with right sides together so that you have a 5" by 6" piece. Stitch up two sides of the pillow, leaving the folded side not sewn and one end open.

3. After it is cut out and sewn on two sides, launder and dry the cloth without using any fragrance or fabric softener. (Dyes and sizing smells in new cloth can cause headaches.)

4. Turn right side out and place a cotton ball-sized amount of cotton or fiberfill material in the bottom of the cloth "pocket."

5. Add about ½ cup of dream blend and place another small amount of cotton or fiberfill on top. (The padding is to make the pillow softer.)

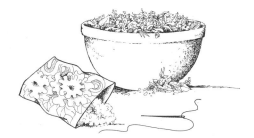

6. Fold over the remaining open end and sew shut by hand with a running stitch. Your dream pillow is now ready to give as a gift or to place inside your pillowcase.

Using the Dream Pillow

People who claim they don't dream are often the ones who are most impressed when they first use a dream pillow because they realize they *have* been dreaming but are just not remembering their dreams. And people who say they never dream in color also often report pleasing results using dream blends.

How long will a dream pillow last? I've used one dream pillow for several years, others for only a few months. Dream pillows seem to work best if I use one for about ten days, then put it away for about that long. I keep mine in a plastic zip bag, so that it stays away from other fragrances. Then I take it back out of the bag and place it inside my pillowcase.

Do dream pillows work for everyone? Most people react to fragrances in pleasant ways. The people who have had the least reaction are heavy smokers, elderly people, and those who use excessive amounts of cologne or perfume; all seem to have desensitized noses. But for most people, fragrance unlocks pleasant memories that play out in their dreams in delightful ways.

Can you dream of something that's not in your memory? In my opinion, yes. The first time I used Inspiring Creativity, I dreamed I was a pirate. I've never even been on a ship, but it was a wonderful experience in the dream.

Should everyone use dream pillows? If you are overly sensitive or allergic to any plants, herbs, or flowers, you should be careful when using a dream blend. If you sneeze or have an allergic reaction to a dream pillow in a waking state, then don't use one in your regular pillow. But for most people, dream pillows are a very enjoyable, fun-filled experience.

Keeping a Dream Log

If you want to be systematic about deciding how effective dream pillows are for you, consider keeping a dream log or simple dream diary. To do that, you need only a little pad or notebook and a pen or pencil. Place the pad on a night table, right where you can reach it while still in bed. You might want to start keeping your dream log a week or more before trying your dream pillow. And it doesn't need to be

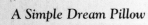

A Simple Dream Pillow

You can use a 3- by 5-inch cotton drawstring bag for your dream pillow if you want something really simple. Place 1/4 to 1/2 cup of the herbs in the bag, draw the strings closed, and tie.

written well, or even in any order beyond quickly scribbled notes. Three or four words will jog your memory later, when you are fully awake.

Immediately upon waking — while you're still groggy — write down your memories of your dream. People usually forget their dreams by the time they've gotten to the bathroom. Most likely, unless you are already a dream log keeper, you'll forget to write anything the first few mornings, remembering only when you notice the pad of paper or when you look into the mirror. But keep trying, and after a couple of days you'll get in the habit of writing something immediately upon waking. You'll likely be surprised to find over time that you have been dreaming, just forgetting the dreams quickly.

Once you've gotten in the practice of keeping the dream log, introduce your dream pillow to your sleep. Your dreams should change over the next several nights and your dream log will reflect that.

Dream Blends vs. Potpourri

Dream blends are very different from potpourri. Dream blends do not contain fragrance oils or essential oils. I never recommend using any kind of oils or fixatives in dream blends; the results are just too unpredictable. And in the case of fragrance or potpourri oils, as the oils evaporate, they change aromas, often causing unpleasant results in the dream.

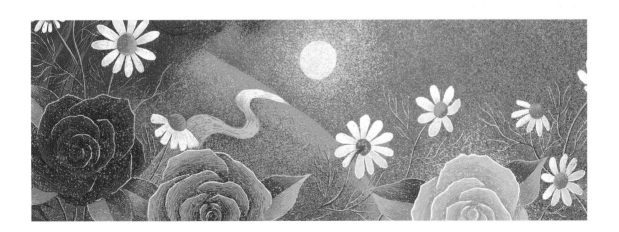

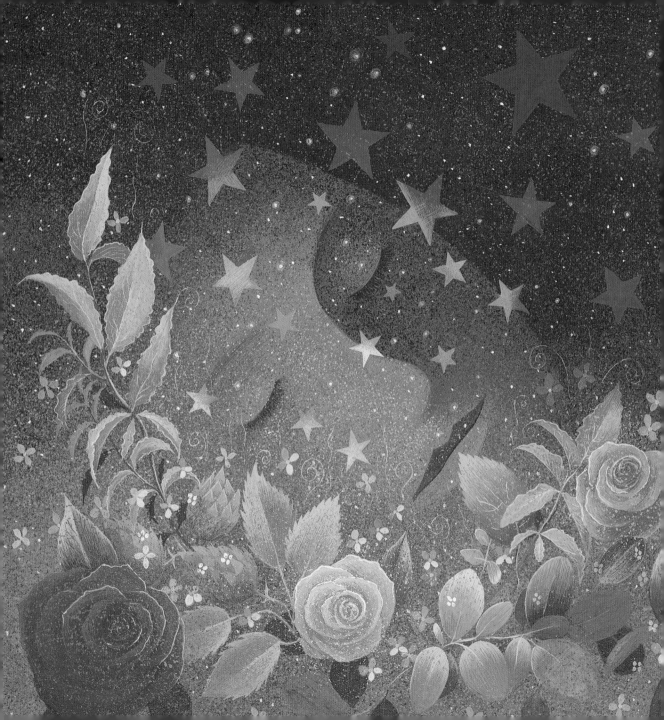

Five Stress-Reducing, Relaxing Dream Blends

Stress from work, family activities, and everyday worries can upset sleeping patterns. These blends won't remove the reasons for the stress, but they often will give a better quality of sleep by preventing unpleasant dreams. The herbs used in stress-reducing blends are those that have been found to help us relax, to give a feeling of safety, and to keep nightmares away.

Restful Sleep

Imagine a soft, billowing comforter, drifting peacefully on a warm breeze. Let yourself float back to childhood, when the soft comforter was the safest place on earth, a place with no worries and all your needs fulfilled.

¼ cup lavender flowers
¼ cup mugwort
¼ cup sweet hops

Stress-Reducing Rest

When I'm drifting off to sleep and want to quiet the dialogue of the day's work in my head, I sometimes like to think of a butterfly's whisper; so quiet, barely heard, still softly drifting on the air.

½ cup sweet hops
½ cup mugwort
⅛ cup sweet marjoram

Peaceful Slumber

I have heard that eating pizza or barbecued ribs late at night can cause nightmares. Perhaps, but not on an ongoing basis. Stress, fear, and worry are the common causes of nightmares. The herbs in this blend should be helpful in easing nightmares and allowing a better night's sleep.

¼ cup roses or rose petals
¼ cup rosemary
¼ cup lavender flowers
¼ cup sweet hops

Hops

are easy to grow in your garden, but they need lots of space. You can easily train them on a trellis. They will climb up to twenty feet or more, then sprout up from the roots. The paperlike greenish flower clusters are the part used. Some recovering alcoholics don't like using hops in their dream blend because it evokes reminders of drinking (bitter hops varieties are an ingredient in beer making).

Rosemary

can be grown as a patio plant; in warm climates (zone 7 or higher), grow it outside. An evergreen shrub, rosemary can be harvested again and again. Hang up the stems to dry, then remove the leaves. Rosemary adds warmth to a dream, along with a feeling of safety. It is said that people in areas of the Mediterranean, where rosemary is native, used to spread out their laundry to dry over rosemary bushes, and that the fragrance left in the laundry brought about peaceful sleep.

To Help You Relax

Sometimes a cup of chamomile tea or a cup of warm milk with honey before bedtime can help you relax.

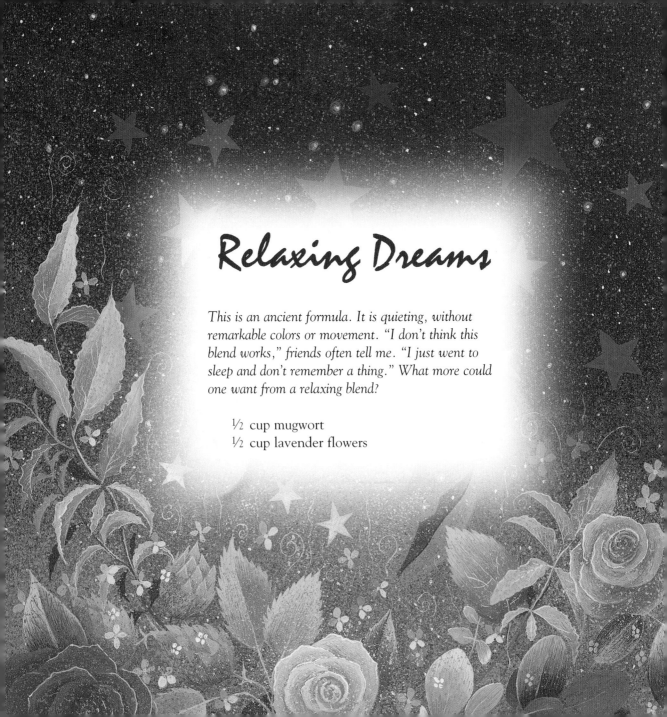

Relaxing Dreams

This is an ancient formula. It is quieting, without remarkable colors or movement. "I don't think this blend works," friends often tell me. "I just went to sleep and don't remember a thing." What more could one want from a relaxing blend?

½ cup mugwort
½ cup lavender flowers

Lavender

is used to ease headaches and to reduce the feelings of stress. Gather lavender flowers just as they are coming into bloom. Cut the stems back to the main cluster of leaves and tie about a dozen stems together. Hang them to dry. Rub the flowers between your thumb and forefinger to remove them from the stem. You may use the stems, but they can poke through the cloth unless you chop them up into ¼-inch or smaller pieces.

Mugwort

is the only artemisia that I know to be useful in dream blends. It has been claimed for centuries to help people remember their dreams, but other plants in that family can cause nightmares and headaches. Mugwort is a strong perennial and you can grow it easily in your garden, but it may become invasive. Place it at the back of a perennial border where its frilly, gray-green leaves and height — it can reach four feet high — will serve as a beautiful backdrop for colorful blooming plants.

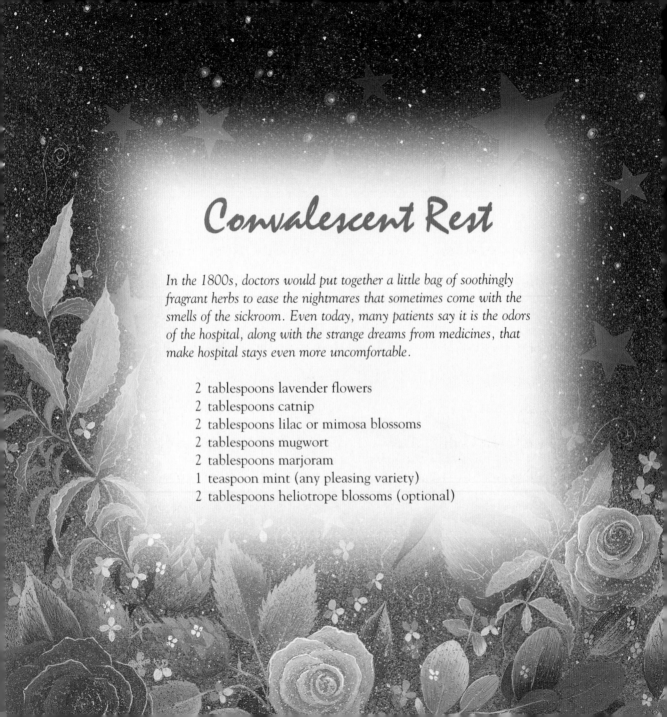

Convalescent Rest

In the 1800s, doctors would put together a little bag of soothingly fragrant herbs to ease the nightmares that sometimes come with the smells of the sickroom. Even today, many patients say it is the odors of the hospital, along with the strange dreams from medicines, that make hospital stays even more uncomfortable.

2 tablespoons lavender flowers
2 tablespoons catnip
2 tablespoons lilac or mimosa blossoms
2 tablespoons mugwort
2 tablespoons marjoram
1 teaspoon mint (any pleasing variety)
2 tablespoons heliotrope blossoms (optional)

Heliotrope

(*Heliotropium* spp.) is a fragrant and relaxing flower. It's used here because the slightly stronger aroma helps combat some of the stronger smells of the sickroom.

Heliotrope is grown from seed or cuttings and is used in borders and annual flower plantings. Gather the flowers throughout the summer and dry them in the same way as you would dry roses.

Lilac

flowers are easy to dry. Cut the woody stems that hold the clusters of blossoms and tie several together to hang in a dry, airy, and dark place. Lilacs can also be laid in a basket and dried in that manner. As soon as the flowers are completely dry and crisp, place them in airtight containers and keep them away from light. The subtle fragrance of lilac flowers will keep for a year or more.

Two Pleasant Dream Blends

Pleasant Dreams Blends give you a boost into a peaceful place.

I like to recall a small clearing in the woods that I found

as a youngster. Giant oaks reached their friendly limbs across,

and the entire ground was carpeted with a beautiful deep

green, velvety-soft moss. A little creek trickled nearby

and I often would take a nap there in the warm sunlight.

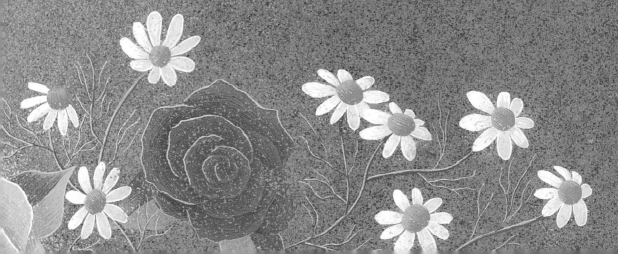

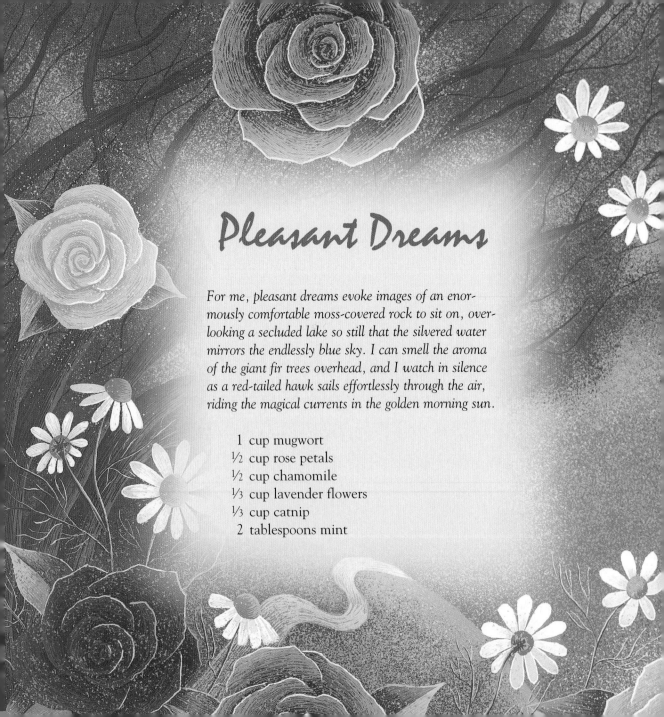

Pleasant Dreams

For me, pleasant dreams evoke images of an enormously comfortable moss-covered rock to sit on, overlooking a secluded lake so still that the silvered water mirrors the endlessly blue sky. I can smell the aroma of the giant fir trees overhead, and I watch in silence as a red-tailed hawk sails effortlessly through the air, riding the magical currents in the golden morning sun.

  1 cup mugwort
  ½ cup rose petals
  ½ cup chamomile
  ⅓ cup lavender flowers
  ⅓ cup catnip
  2 tablespoons mint

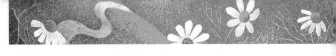
Chamomile

is found in two basic kinds, Roman
(*Chamaemelum nobile*) and German
(*Matricaria chamomilla*, listed in some sources
as *Chamomilla recutita*). This last one, an
easily grown annual reaching about fifteen
inches in height, is the one to use for dream
blends. Roman chamomile grows more like a
short carpet or ground cover and is not as
useful for the purposes here, but you can
combine both kinds if you wish.

Mint

with a good, pleasant fragrance is the best
kind to use. The preferable mint for dream
blends is peppermint or spearmint, but other
kinds work as well. I don't like to use the
mint called pineapple — it smells soapy to
me — but I've used several of the others in
dream blends, including those that are listed
with common names like apple, orange and
lemon.

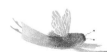

Blending Tip
*This recipe makes enough for five or six dream pillows.
You can cut the amounts in half, but all are so small
that it is just as easy to make the whole amount.*

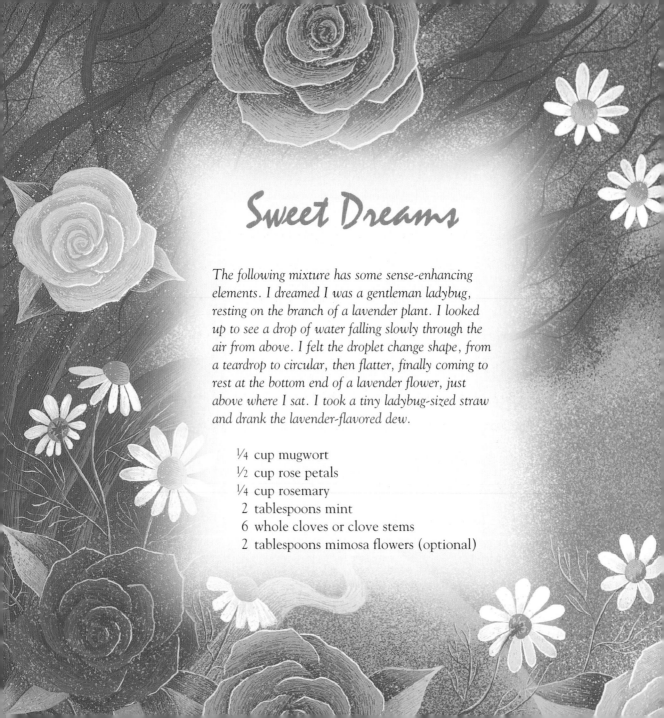

Sweet Dreams

The following mixture has some sense-enhancing elements. I dreamed I was a gentleman ladybug, resting on the branch of a lavender plant. I looked up to see a drop of water falling slowly through the air from above. I felt the droplet change shape, from a teardrop to circular, then flatter, finally coming to rest at the bottom end of a lavender flower, just above where I sat. I took a tiny ladybug-sized straw and drank the lavender-flavored dew.

   ¼ cup mugwort
   ½ cup rose petals
   ¼ cup rosemary
   2 tablespoons mint
   6 whole cloves or clove stems
   2 tablespoons mimosa flowers (optional)

Cloves

add a more exotic, spicy feeling to dreams, especially when used with roses in romantic mixtures. The exotic smell, when combined with flowers, can invoke more complex and exciting dreaming, including more color, possibly more movement, and often more excitement in the plot. Use cloves sparingly; three or four cloves to a blend would be plenty. Whole cloves are the more expensive product, but clove stems can be a good substitute.

Mimosa

flowers are pleasant in this mix, if you have them. Mimosa trees have naturalized in some areas of the country and are still a common backyard tree. Gather the flowers before they drop from the tree and lay them on newspapers, on a cookie sheet, to dry. They have a mild but sweet tropical aroma and can be used in many dream blends.

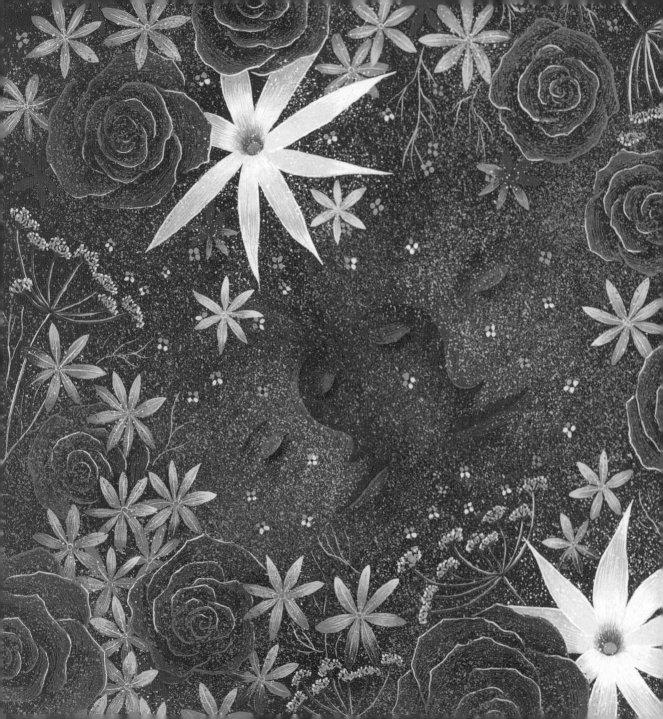

Four Romantic
Dream Blends

The vivid, silken petals of red roses are even more fragrant

in a romantic dream. Our minds build the ideal romantic setting:

Chocolates are more tempting, wines are of a deeper hue,

and the music is perfectly tuned. Romance is a sensual,

sweet, safe, sometimes erotic, always enjoyable place in our

minds that we like to return to again and again.

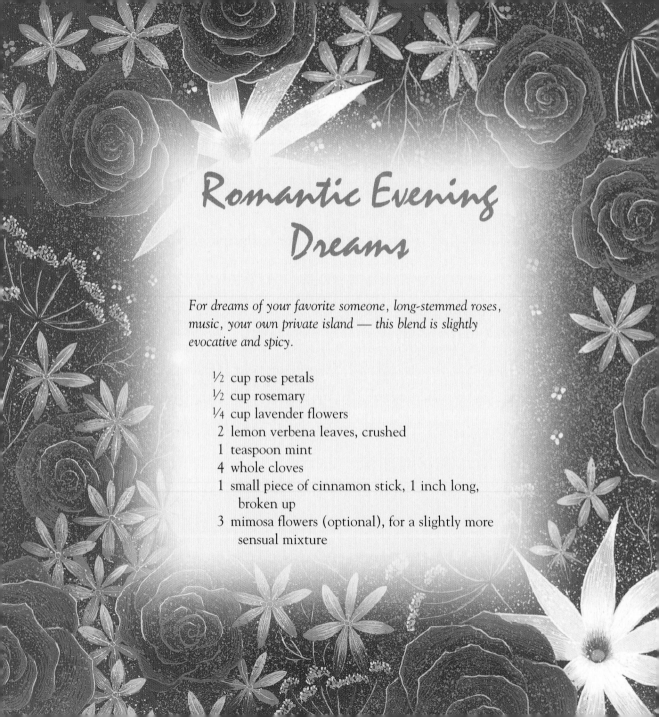

Romantic Evening Dreams

For dreams of your favorite someone, long-stemmed roses, music, your own private island — this blend is slightly evocative and spicy.

  ½ cup rose petals
  ½ cup rosemary
  ¼ cup lavender flowers
  2 lemon verbena leaves, crushed
  1 teaspoon mint
  4 whole cloves
  1 small piece of cinnamon stick, 1 inch long,
     broken up
  3 mimosa flowers (optional), for a slightly more
     sensual mixture

Lemon verbena

is a delightful plant. I grow mine outdoors in the garden, in a moist but sunny spot. In the fall, I dig up the plant, prune back the top and roots if needed, and pot it in a clay container. The following spring, I replant it outdoors and enjoy a bounty of deliciously lemony leaves all season. Not only is this a great dream herb, but I also use the leaves for tea, desserts, and in fruit salads.

Cinnamon,

like cloves, adds some warmth and spice to a blend. Be sure to use real cinnamon if possible, rather than cassia, a related plant with a similar, but fainter, fragrance. Real cinnamon has a pungent, spicy aroma; its less expensive cousin is a poor substitute. You can grow cinnamon as a potted plant. The leaves will also have the pleasant, but milder fragrance of the mature tree, and can be used in several different dream blends as well.

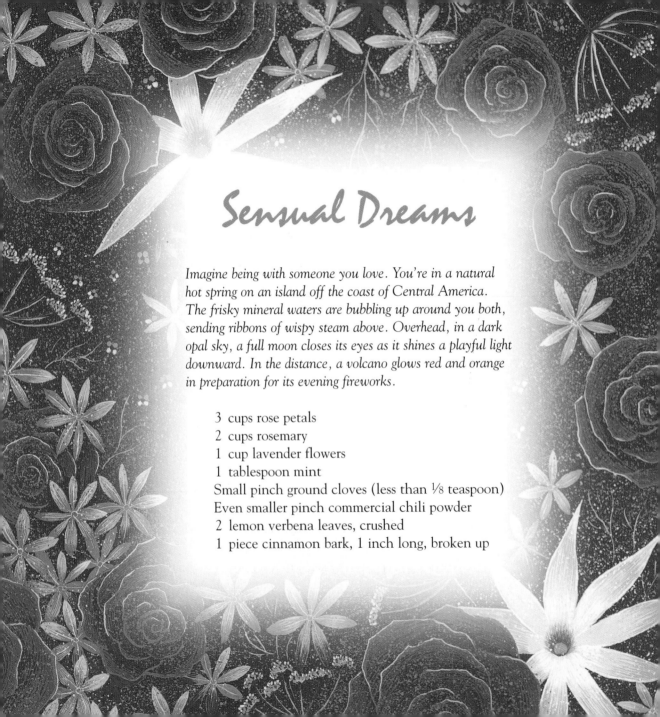

Sensual Dreams

Imagine being with someone you love. You're in a natural hot spring on an island off the coast of Central America. The frisky mineral waters are bubbling up around you both, sending ribbons of wispy steam above. Overhead, in a dark opal sky, a full moon closes its eyes as it shines a playful light downward. In the distance, a volcano glows red and orange in preparation for its evening fireworks.

3 cups rose petals
2 cups rosemary
1 cup lavender flowers
1 tablespoon mint
Small pinch ground cloves (less than ⅛ teaspoon)
Even smaller pinch commercial chili powder
2 lemon verbena leaves, crushed
1 piece cinnamon bark, 1 inch long, broken up

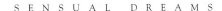

Chili powder?

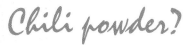

Sure. It's made from ground-up herb plants, including several kinds of peppers, cumin, allspice, oregano, and garlic. The addition of a very small amount gives a boost to the sensuousness, the exotic feeling of romance in this mix. It will add intensified color, especially if mint is included in the mix, along with a dimension of intensity. You may find yourself playing out fantasies in dreams from just the tiniest hint of this spicy herb blend.

Wishing for Love
An old folk formula for love instructs you to place lavender under the pillow while thinking of your wish for love. If you do this the last thing before going to bed, any dreams during the night should come true.

Amorous Dreams

Friends have described their dreams after using the following blend as full of color in vividly romantic settings. One friend said, "It was like we were two feathers, floating on a spring breeze, crossing paths, touching, drifting over moonlit beaches."

2 tablespoons sweet hops flowers
2 tablespoons calendula petals
2 tablespoons rose petals
2 tablespoons jasmine flowers
1 tablespoon catnip
1 tablespoon marjoram
2 teaspoons lemon verbena leaves
2 teaspoons lavender flowers
2 teaspoons mint

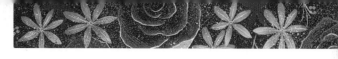

Calendula

is added here to balance the effects of the
other herbs. Also known as pot marigold, this
is an easily grown annual. Plant the seed in
spring or in late summer, as it prefers moder-
ately cool temperatures, and harvest the flowers all during blooming time. Snap off the
flower heads just as they are fully open and
toss them into a basket to dry. The recipe
calls for petals, but you can just as easily use
the whole dried flower head.

Marjoram,

also called sweet marjoram, is a sweet, sort of
pine-scented member of the oregano family.
I've found it to be relaxing in dream blends,
but marjoram adds some spice and comple-
ments the more exotic fragrance of jasmine.
Marjoram is simple to grow in the garden as
an annual from seed. Folklore asserts that
marjoram by itself might make you dream of
playful fairies.

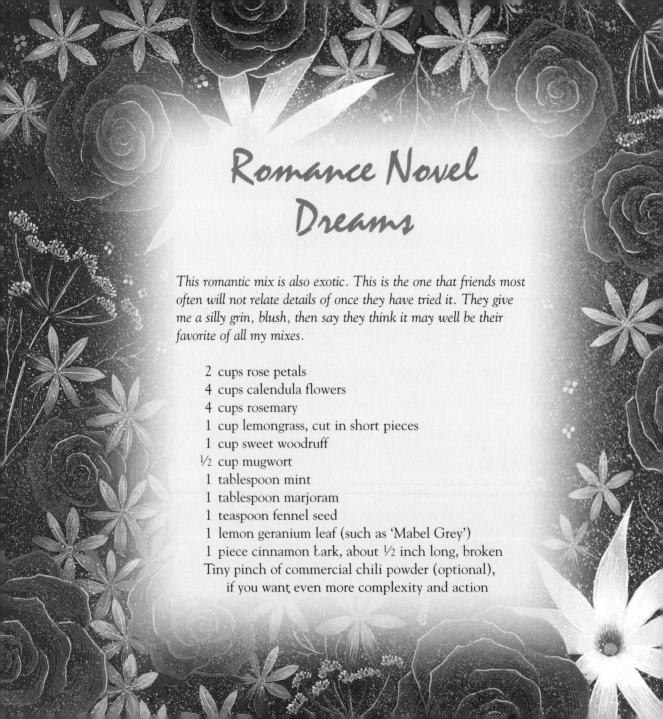

Romance Novel Dreams

This romantic mix is also exotic. This is the one that friends most often will not relate details of once they have tried it. They give me a silly grin, blush, then say they think it may well be their favorite of all my mixes.

2 cups rose petals
4 cups calendula flowers
4 cups rosemary
1 cup lemongrass, cut in short pieces
1 cup sweet woodruff
½ cup mugwort
1 tablespoon mint
1 tablespoon marjoram
1 teaspoon fennel seed
1 lemon geranium leaf (such as 'Mabel Grey')
1 piece cinnamon bark, about ½ inch long, broken
Tiny pinch of commercial chili powder (optional),
    if you want even more complexity and action

Lemon geranium

(*Pelargonium crispum*) isn't listed in the official list of dream blend plants in chapter 1, but it's worth ordering from a mail-order house if you haven't grown it before; it's an important ingredient in this blend. The Pelargonium family is large, with lots of different scented geraniums, such as orange, rose, lemon, and peppermint. My favorite lemon-scented varieties are 'Mabel Grey' and 'Prince Ruppert'. Their fragrance is pleasantly lemon and spice.

Fennel seed

(*Foeniculum vulgare*) is another ingredient not commonly used, and not listed in the introductory plant list. In this mix it adds lightness — a feeling of flying or leaping with joy. It's the same fennel seed you'll find in the grocery store, and it's usually used to spice up a recipe. Plant a few of the seeds and grow your own fennel plant in the garden, too.

Blending Tip

This recipe makes enough for about a dozen pillows, but if you reduce the amounts, you will upset the balance of the small amounts of lemon geranium, fennel, and cinnamon. I recommend keeping the amounts true to the recipe and giving some away to friends. They make great valentine gifts!

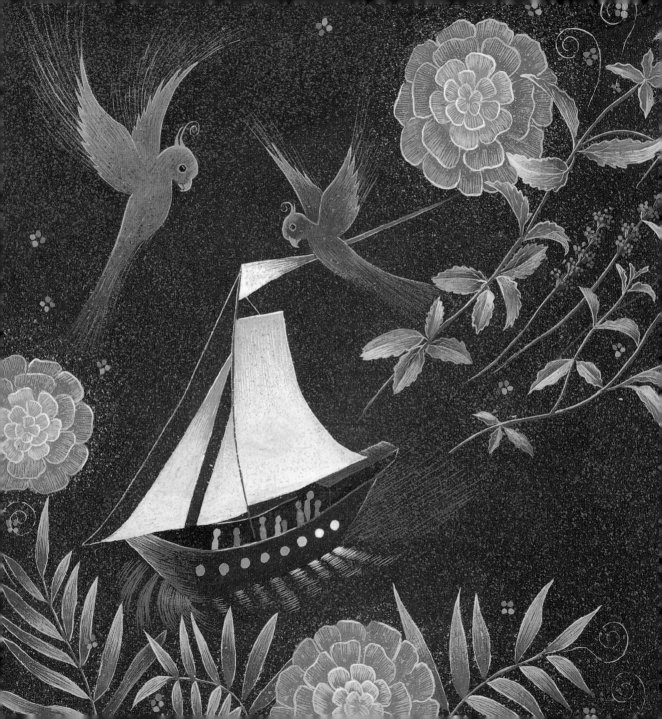

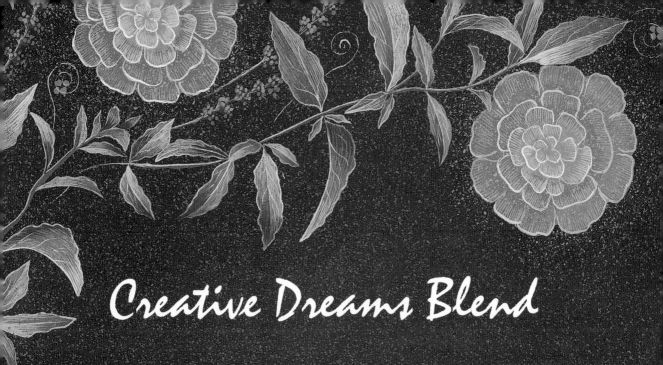

Creative Dreams Blend

This blend provides great color and movement.

In one dream I was a pirate on an elegant black ship,

sailing on an agate blue sea. I remember the colorful costumes,

the brilliant sky, the crisp white sails, even a green-and-red

parrot that was energetically singing. I felt I could write

about the sea, or paint a picture, or portray a pirate

with complete accuracy.

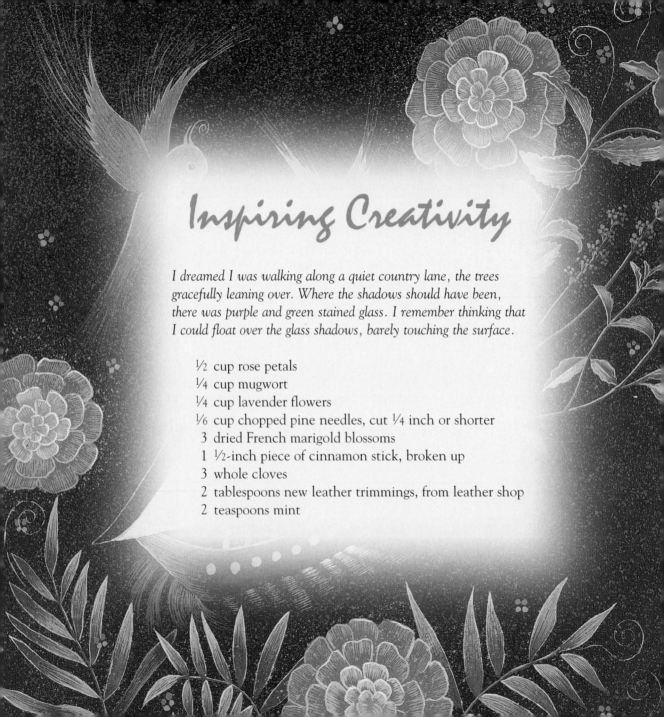

Inspiring Creativity

I dreamed I was walking along a quiet country lane, the trees gracefully leaning over. Where the shadows should have been, there was purple and green stained glass. I remember thinking that I could float over the glass shadows, barely touching the surface.

½ cup rose petals
¼ cup mugwort
¼ cup lavender flowers
⅙ cup chopped pine needles, cut ¼ inch or shorter
3 dried French marigold blossoms
1 ½-inch piece of cinnamon stick, broken up
3 whole cloves
2 tablespoons new leather trimmings, from leather shop
2 teaspoons mint

French marigolds

(Tagetes patula) are generally not used in dream blends because they are too strongly scented and in large quantities can cause headaches or nightmares. In this blend, however, using just three whole blossoms (the yellow and green parts) enhances the colors in the dream. It is the slightly bitter quality of the marigold blossom that allows the fragrance of the pine needles and leather trimmings to prompt the mind to seek out new and exciting settings.

Pine needles

give a dream blend an outdoors texture. You can easily dry your own pine needles for this project; any kind of pine will do. Cut a small branch, one with a limb about the size of a toothpick. Gather the needles together between the thumb and fingers of one hand. With scissors in the other hand, start clipping on the stem end, working your way up onto the needles until you have snipped everything — including the stem — into very small pieces.

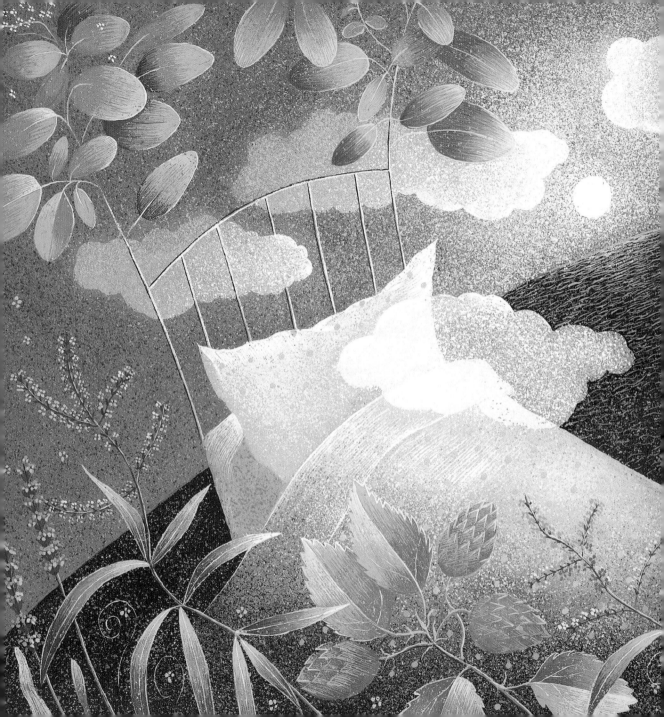

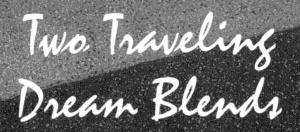

Two Traveling Dream Blends

These blends are meant to give quiet rest, a familiar scent, and

peacefulness to the traveler, in order to inspire confidence

and ensure the fullest enjoyment of the trip. This security may

come in the form of being a child again, feeling protected

by parents who love you and by the knowledge

that there is no place on earth safer than your bed.

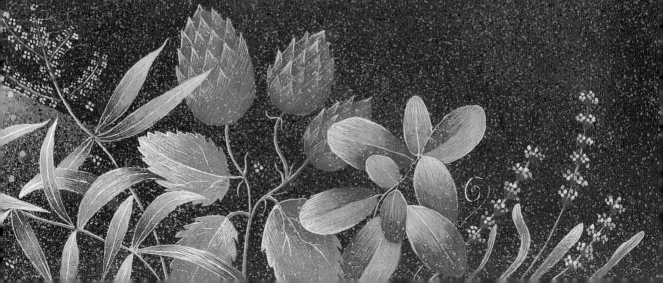

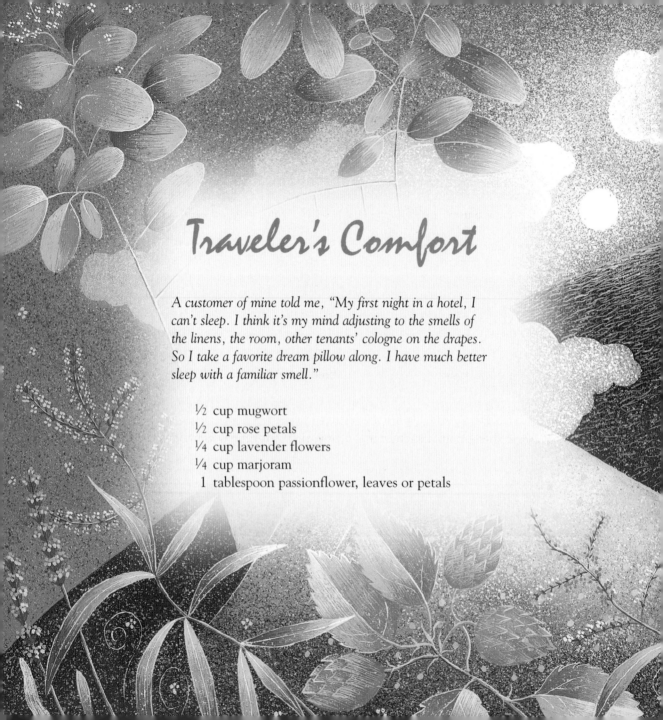

Traveler's Comfort

A customer of mine told me, "My first night in a hotel, I can't sleep. I think it's my mind adjusting to the smells of the linens, the room, other tenants' cologne on the drapes. So I take a favorite dream pillow along. I have much better sleep with a familiar smell."

½ cup mugwort
½ cup rose petals
¼ cup lavender flowers
¼ cup marjoram
1 tablespoon passionflower, leaves or petals

Passionflower

is a vine grown for its frilly, colored flowers. The leaves and flowers are used as a sedative. Here's an easy way to dry passionflower. Put several flowers and leaves in a small paper bag. Fold the top and secure with a paper clip. Place the bag on the dashboard of your car during the day in the heat of summer. As soon as the herbs have dried (this will take about one day), store them in an airtight container in a darkened place until you're ready to mix your dream blend.

Roses

come in many varieties, but the best ones to use in dream blends are the fragrant varieties of shrub or antique roses. Many of these date back several centuries, unchanged, sturdy and deliciously fragrant. The most ineffective roses to use for dream blends are tea roses. These are bred for show, with little regard to fragrance.

Gather roses for drying during midmorning, right after the dew has dried. Scatter the petals into a little basket and place it in a warm, airy, dark place. With your hands, stir the petals every day until they are dried.

Blending Tip
Place this pillow in a plastic zipper bag before packing it in your suitcase.

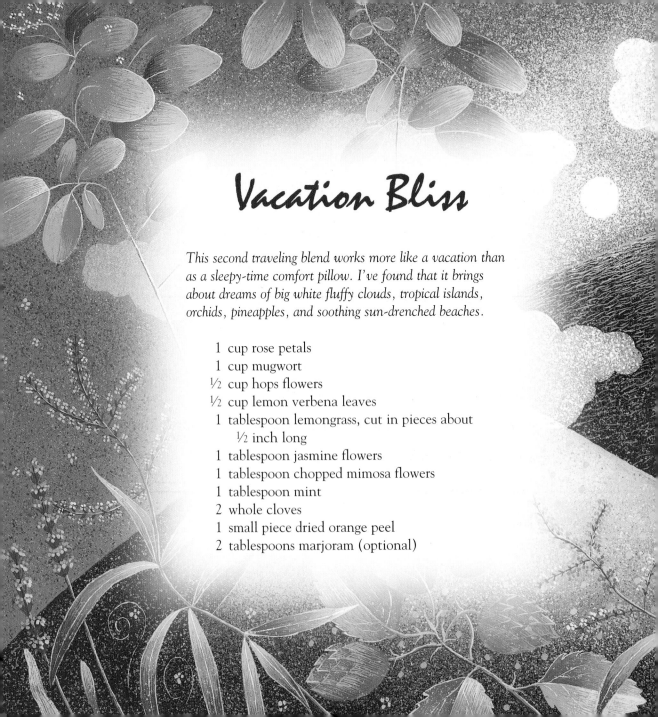

Vacation Bliss

This second traveling blend works more like a vacation than
as a sleepy-time comfort pillow. I've found that it brings
about dreams of big white fluffy clouds, tropical islands,
orchids, pineapples, and soothing sun-drenched beaches.

  1 cup rose petals
  1 cup mugwort
  ½ cup hops flowers
  ½ cup lemon verbena leaves
  1 tablespoon lemongrass, cut in pieces about
     ½ inch long
  1 tablespoon jasmine flowers
  1 tablespoon chopped mimosa flowers
  1 tablespoon mint
  2 whole cloves
  1 small piece dried orange peel
  2 tablespoons marjoram (optional)

Lemongrass,

found in Oriental produce stores, is a fresh, bulblike grass. It likes moist to wet soil and full sun. To harvest lemongrass, snip off leaf blades and cut them up, then dry them in the shade.

In the fall I cut back the lemongrass, dig up the clump, pot it, and move it inside. In the spring, I remove it from the pot and replant it in the garden, where it quickly grows into lush and attractive, three-foot-tall, light green grass.

Jasmine

flowers are a bit harder to find unless you have a greenhouse and can grow them yourself, or live in a warm climate. The flowers are available in many whole foods stores that sell herbs in bulk or by the scoop, or from mail-order suppliers. Fragrance researchers suggest that jasmine is one of the most sensual fragrances for women.

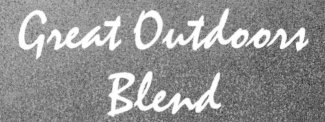

Great Outdoors Blend

Once I dreamed I was a red-tailed hawk.

I remember the sensation of sailing through the air,

well above the treetops. I saw the ground in every

detail from above, my eyes keen and sharp. I felt the air

as it flowed softly over my feathers. I was strong and

confident; this was my air, my sky, my realm.

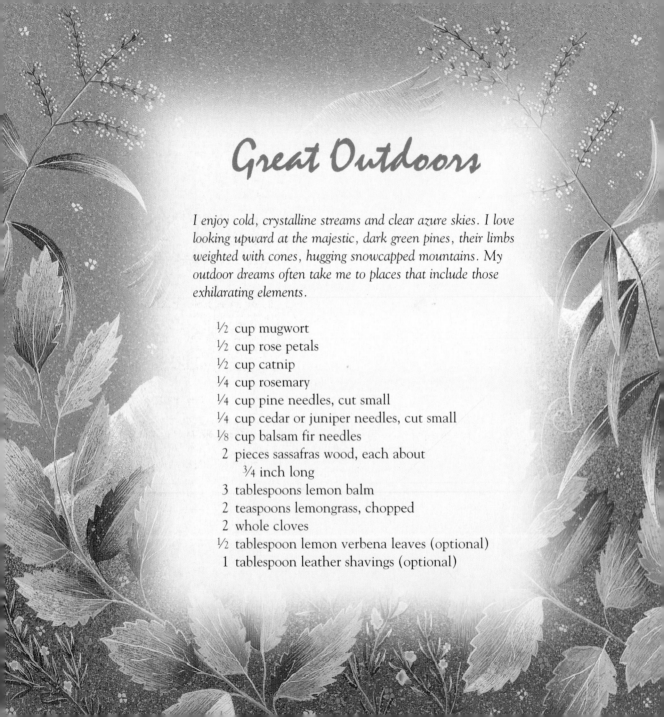

Great Outdoors

I enjoy cold, crystalline streams and clear azure skies. I love looking upward at the majestic, dark green pines, their limbs weighted with cones, hugging snowcapped mountains. My outdoor dreams often take me to places that include those exhilarating elements.

½ cup mugwort
½ cup rose petals
½ cup catnip
¼ cup rosemary
¼ cup pine needles, cut small
¼ cup cedar or juniper needles, cut small
⅛ cup balsam fir needles
2 pieces sassafras wood, each about
   ¾ inch long
3 tablespoons lemon balm
2 teaspoons lemongrass, chopped
2 whole cloves
½ tablespoon lemon verbena leaves (optional)
1 tablespoon leather shavings (optional)

Cedar and balsam fir

needles add a woodsy feeling to the dream. If you don't have those, use any other varieties of juniper and fir that are available to you. Snip them finely and dry them for several days until they are brittle and break apart easily. Use cedar sparingly, about two teaspoonfuls per pillow. Cedar berries can also be used this way.

Sassafras wood

isn't listed in the introductory plant list, but it is useful in this mix to add a spicy, outdoorsy feeling. Sassafras tea bags are still available in gourmet food and whole foods stores. Or you can snip a small limb or root from your own tree if you have one. I don't recommend using sassafras oil, which is quite different and gives unpredictable results.

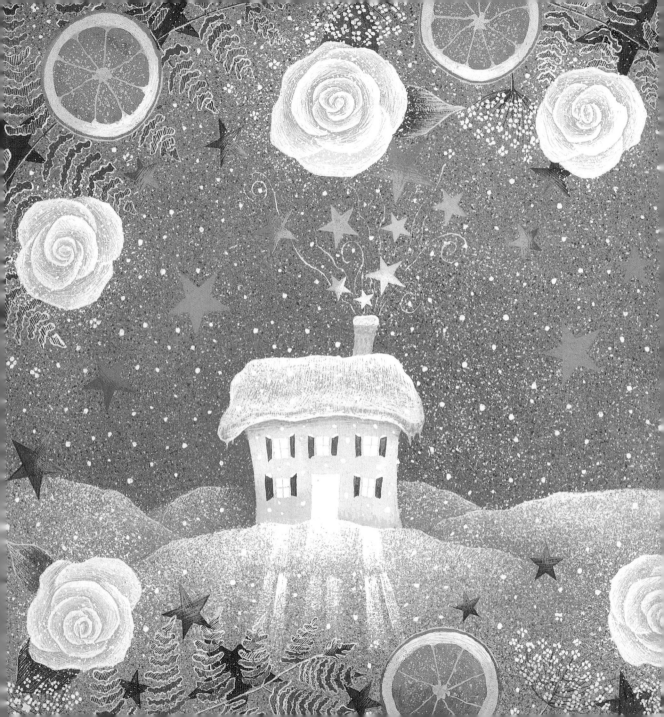

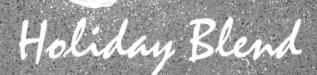

Holiday Blend

My dreams of the holidays are always of fluffy drifts of snow

and a two-story white house with green shutters.

There are smells of baking bread and spicy desserts, and the

aroma of fresh evergreens. Bowls of oranges, apples,

and homemade candies grace tables in every room.

Candles glow, my grandmother plays the piano,

and everyone gathers around to sing.

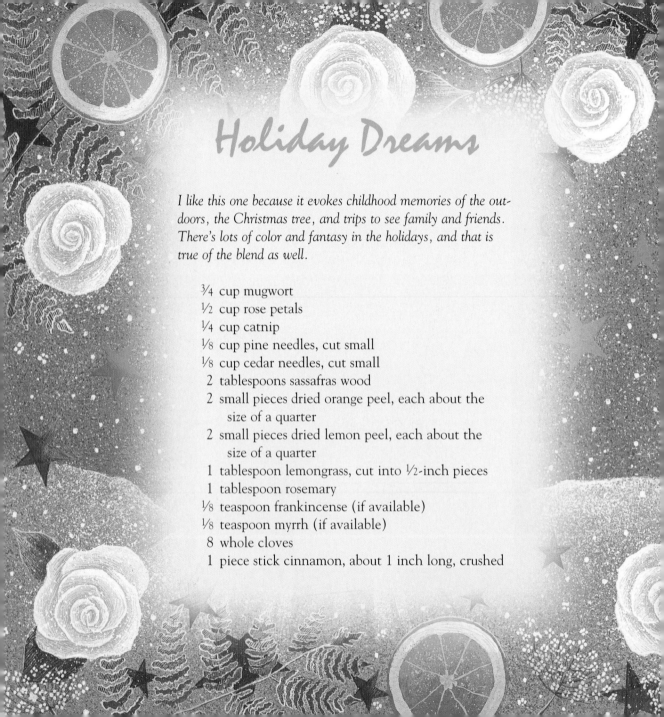

Holiday Dreams

I like this one because it evokes childhood memories of the out-
doors, the Christmas tree, and trips to see family and friends.
There's lots of color and fantasy in the holidays, and that is
true of the blend as well.

¾ cup mugwort
½ cup rose petals
¼ cup catnip
⅛ cup pine needles, cut small
⅛ cup cedar needles, cut small
2 tablespoons sassafras wood
2 small pieces dried orange peel, each about the
   size of a quarter
2 small pieces dried lemon peel, each about the
   size of a quarter
1 tablespoon lemongrass, cut into ½-inch pieces
1 tablespoon rosemary
⅛ teaspoon frankincense (if available)
⅛ teaspoon myrrh (if available)
8 whole cloves
1 piece stick cinnamon, about 1 inch long, crushed

Frankincense and myrrh

are tree resins, and are generally used as incense (burnt on self-activating charcoal disks). The incense has a faint odor. Crush with a spoon or in a blender, or buy the powdered resin.

Frankincense and myrrh were once as precious as gold. You'll recall from the Bible that the Christ child was given gifts of gold, frankincense, and myrrh. Gold was for support of the family; the incense was a commodity reserved for kings. They are ancient aromas and round out this blend for dreams of the wonders of the season.

Citrus peel,

including lemon, orange, grapefruit, and tangerine, gives dreams an energetic tone, as well as evoking lots of playful memories. Used sparingly, citrus combines with spicy fragrances to evoke pleasant and colorful dreams.

You can buy dried orange or lemon peel, but I prefer the less expensive alternative, buying the oranges and first eating them. Then lay the peelings in little baskets and put them where the air from the furnace blows across them. In less than a week, you will have fragrant, freshly dried orange peels — and have gotten your daily allowance of vitamin C.

Blending Tip

This mixture has many of the fragrances of an old-time Christmas. It's a complex mix, and will provide enough blend to give to friends. The recipe makes five or six dream pillows if you use about 4 tablespoonfuls for each.

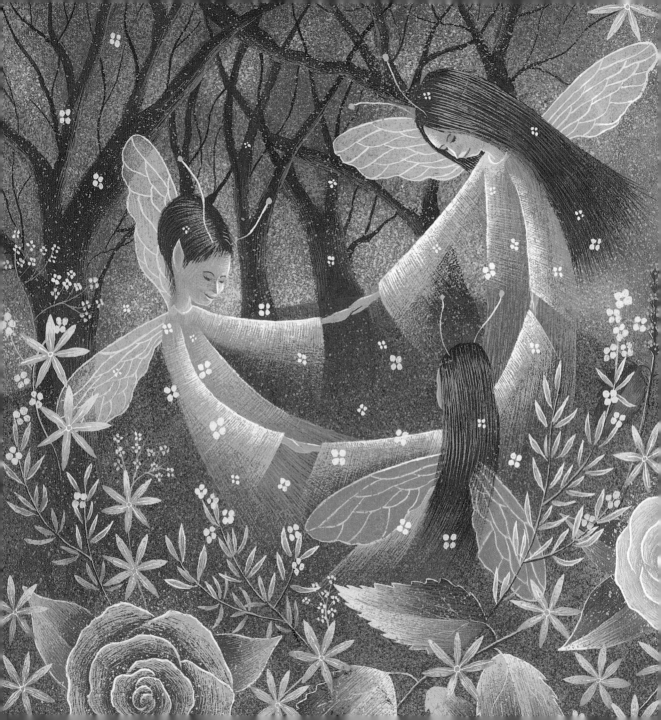

Prophecy Blend

A number of herbs have a long history of use in dream

pillows, and are said to promote dreams of flying,

dreams of innocence and inspiration. Perhaps you'll

dream of fairies, their gossamer gold wings unfolding

as they tell stories of emerald forests and unicorns,

times when elves lived all around, when people

and nature still spoke the same language.

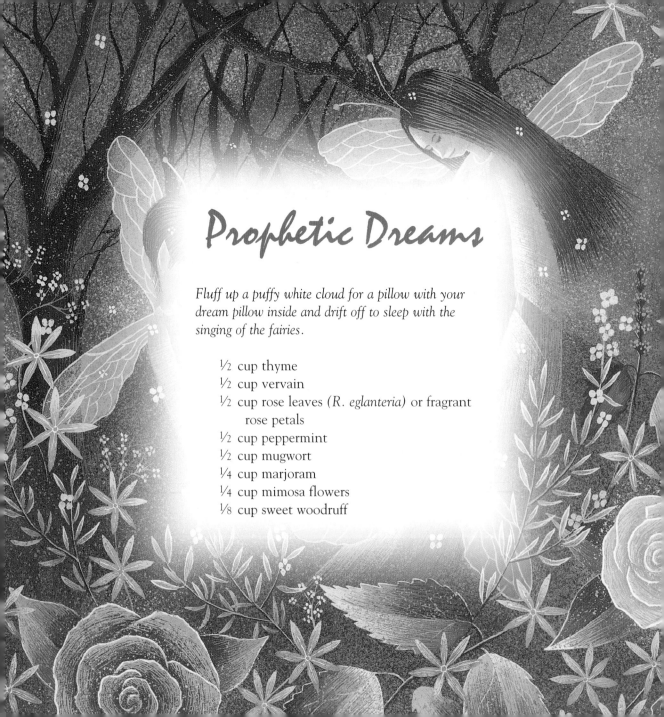

Prophetic Dreams

Fluff up a puffy white cloud for a pillow with your dream pillow inside and drift off to sleep with the singing of the fairies.

½ cup thyme
½ cup vervain
½ cup rose leaves (*R. eglanteria*) or fragrant
    rose petals
½ cup peppermint
½ cup mugwort
¼ cup marjoram
¼ cup mimosa flowers
⅛ cup sweet woodruff

Vervain

(*Verbena officinalis*) has lots of ties to magic and prophetic dreams. It's a native plant, with variations found in many parts of the United States. (Consult a wildflower book for proper identification.) You can gather both the flowers and leaves for this. You won't notice much of an odor, but it doesn't take a lot in a dream blend to be effective. According to folklore, vervain keeps away nightmares and gives relaxing sleep.

Sweet woodruff

(*Asperula odorata*) was believed centuries ago to be useful to protect the dreamer from nightmares. Protection from nightmares is another way of describing pleasant sleep. Sweet woodruff is better known today as the flavoring in May wine and as a shade-loving ground cover, easy to grow under trees in your yard.

To See the Fairies

Folklore contends that wearing thyme allows you to see fairies in the moonlight. Thyme is generally thought of as relaxing when used with roses, but it can be slightly stimulating and color-enhancing when combined with sweeter fragrances such as mimosa and sweet woodruff. Thyme helps create feelings of lightness and may promote airy dreams of flying.

Resources

Bluejay Gardens
Route 2, Box 196
Haskell, OK 74436
(309) 385-2589
Plants, herbs, wedding herbs.
Price list available on request.

Dry Creek Herb Farm
13935 Dry Creek Road
Auburn, CA 95602
(916) 878-2441
Mail-order catalog.

Greenfield Herb Garden
P.O. Box 9
Shipshewana, IN 46565
(219) 768-7110
(800) 831-0504
Fax (219) 768-7092
Plants, seeds, supplies, bulk herbs.
Mail-order catalog.

Jean's Greens
119 Sulphur Spring Road
Newport, NY 13416
(888) 845-8327
Mail-order catalog.

Long Creek Herbs
Jim Long's company
Route 4, Box 730
Oak Grove, AR 72660
Phone and Fax orders:
(417) 779-5450
www.longcreekherbs.com
Supplier of dream pillows, dream
blends, dream pillow supplies, and
bulk herbs. Catalog $2, refundable
with first order.

Moutain Rose Herbs
20818 High Street
North San Juan, CA 95960
(800) 879-3337
Fax (530) 292-9138
Mail-order catalog.

Nichols Garden Nursery
1190 North Pacific Highway
Albany, OR 97321-4598
www.pacificharbor.com/nichols/
Herb plants (many varieties of
hops), seed, bulk herbs, supplies.
Mail-order catalog.

Our Family's Herbs & Such
702 Llano
Pasadena, TX 77504
(800) 441-1230
Bulk herbs and supplies.
Mail-order catalog.

Pinetree Garden Seeds
Box 300
New Gloucester, ME 04260
(207) 926-3400
Herb seeds in small packets,
books, bulbs. Mail-order catalog.

Richter's
357 Highway 47
Goodwood, ON
LOC 1A0 Canada
(416) 640-6677
Herb seed and plants. Mail-order
catalog.

Rosemary House
120 South Market Street
Mechanicsburg, PA 17055
(717) 697-5111
Seeds, plants, supplies, books.
Mail-order catalog, $2.

Shady Acres Herb Farm
7815 Highway 212
Chaska, MN 55318
(612) 466-3391
www.shadyacres.com
Herb plants and books.
Mail-order catalog, $2.

Other Storey Titles You Will Enjoy

At Home with Herbs: Inspiring Ideas for Cooking, Crafts, Decorating, and Cosmetics, by Jane Newdick. 224 pages. Hardcover. ISBN 0-88266-886-2.

Creating Fairy Garden Fragrances, by Linda Gannon. 64 pages. Hardcover. ISBN 1-58017-076-5.

Growing Your Herb Business, by Bertha Reppert. 192 pages. Paperback. ISBN 0-88266-612-6.

The Herbal Body Book: A Natural Approach to Healthier Hair, Skin, and Nails, by Stephanie Tourles. 128 pages. Paperback. ISBN 0-88266-880-3.

The Herb Gardener: A Guide for All Seasons, by Susan McClure. 240 pages. Hardcover. ISBN 0-88266-910-9. Paperback: ISBN 0-88266-873-0.

The Herbal Home Remedy Book: Simple Recipes for Tinctures, Teas, Salves, Tonics, and Syrups, by Joyce A. Wardwell. 176 pages. Paperback. ISBN 1-58017-016-1.

The Herbal Home Spa: Naturally Refreshing Wraps, Rubs, Lotions, Masks, Oils, and Scrubs, by Greta Breedlove. 208 pages. Paperback. ISBN 1-58107-005-6.

Herbal Treasures: Inspiring Month-by-Month Projects for Gardening, Cooking, and Crafts, by Phyllis V. Shaudys. 320 pages. Paperback. ISBN 0-88266-618-5.

Making Bentwood Trellises, Arbors, Gates & Fences, by Jim Long. 160 pages. Paperback. ISBN 1-58017-051-X.

These and other Storey books are available at your bookstore, herb shop, garden center, or directly from Storey Books, Schoolhouse Road, Pownal, Vermont 05261, or by calling 1-800-441-5700. Or visit our web site at www.storey.com.